Skin Care:
25 Homemade Natural Recipes Made of Herbs and Essential Oils

This document is geared towards providing exact and reliable information in regards to the topic and issue covered. The publication is sold with the idea that the publisher is not required to render accounting, officially permitted, or otherwise, qualified services. If advice is necessary, legal or professional, a practiced individual in the profession should be ordered.

- From a Declaration of Principles which was accepted and approved equally by a Committee of the American Bar Association and a Committee of Publishers and Associations.

Table of content

Introduction

There you are, standing in another beauty store, trying to find just what you need for your skin. It's summer, so you have to worry about sunburn and dry skin. Or perhaps it's winter, and you have to worry about dry skin on top of dry skin.

You know what you want. You need something that is organic, something that is good for you, and something you love the scent of. Nothing that is second best will do, you have to have the best of the best and leave the rest to the rest.

So what do you do?

As you browse the shelves, you find item after item that claims to be what you want, but you just don't know if it's organic, if it's all natural, or if it's really worth the price. You want to do what is best for your skin, but how do you decide what you are going to spend on a bottle of product when you know you have other bills to pay?

When it comes to your health, you can't put a price on what you have. You know that your health is more important than anything, but at the same time, you have to consider the other expenses you have in your day. That is why you should get in the habit of making things yourself.

When you make your own skin care products, you not only know for sure what is going into them, but you know without a doubt what you are putting on your body. You know you can rest assured knowing they are healthy options and that you are only going to get the good from using them.

This gives you the assurance you need to use them with confidence whenever you like, whether it is in the heat of summer, the cool of winter, or if you are going to use them every day no matter what the weather is like.

This book is going to show you how to make your own skin care products, and how to keep your lifestyle as healthy as you want it to be. No guesswork, no crazy prices for things you can't pronounce, and no more wondering if you are going to get the help your skin needs while sticking with your skin standards.

This book is everything you need to make it all work, and to make it come together as you need it to. Get ready to dive into the world of clean living, and embrace the all natural skin care regime your body craves.

You'll never go back to the old way of doing things again.

Chapter 1 – Organic Options for Oily Skin

The Perfect Kiss

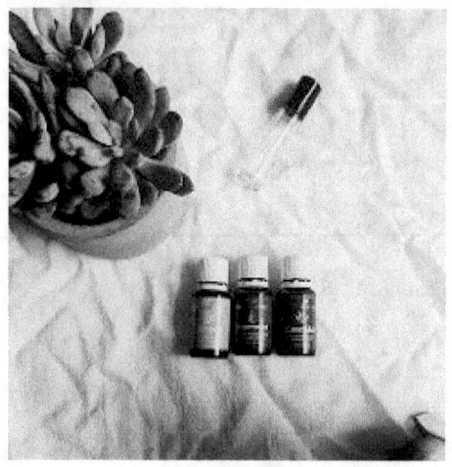

https://www.flickr.com/photos/vanillaandlaceblog/17255454236/in/photolist-shNHnE-8vEXkh-a1XWoX-e2AAik-e2AAbV-79m1GY-79ha7z-oAWCZN-cSWygw-oUfH18-e2GekE-e2Gerw-c6dPw1-c6dQzh-e2AA52-e2AA0H-diH6ED-avi-HH7-c6dQ6J-shNBs0-qMDNKT-mwJpD3-4vgg87-ncFQvr-8vBVVr-8vEXcj-cT8D2J-cSWAe7-0jUBwM-4HcFZL-cTv3Ej-pNGMCN-eUgFX6-cTv2hN-8vBVTe-8vEXjo-c6dNcA-e7gX8o-wEWXTH-G2LbRB-8NwKFG-6zeTxV-s1LFda-6jdUsn-mwFMgM-5nWqne-bosoFP-8vEXd9-8vBWaH-cT8CwW

What you will need:

10 drops neroli oil

5 drops tea tree oil

1 teaspoon organic wild black raspberry leaves

1 teaspoon almond oil

1 teaspoon coconut oil

Directions:

Heat ¼ cup water on the stove until hot, but not boiling. Soak the leaves in this water for 5 minutes.

You can strain out the leaves if you like, or you can leave them in… it's really up to you. I prefer to take them out, as they tend to get too soggy if I don't use all of the treatment at one time, but if you don't mind, leave them in.

Combine the rest of the ingredients in with the water, and carefully stir. You want them all to be as mixed as possible.

Let the mix cool until it is warm, then apply generously to your skin. Massage in and leave on or rinse off.

Store any leftover treatment in an airtight glass jar until you are ready to use again.

Beach Babe

What you will need:

10 drops grapefruit oil

5 drops lemon oil

1 teaspoon dried spruce needles, crushed

1 teaspoon almond oil

1 teaspoon coconut oil

Directions:

Heat ¼ cup water on the stove until hot, but not boiling. Soak the spruce in this water for 5 minutes.

You can strain out the needles if you like, or you can leave them in... it's really up to you. I prefer to take them out, as they tend to get too soggy if I don't use all of the treatment at one time, but if you don't mind, leave them in.

Combine the rest of the ingredients in with the water, and carefully stir. You want them all to be as mixed as possible.

Let the mix cool until it is warm, then apply generously to your skin. Massage in and leave on or rinse off.

Store any leftover treatment in an airtight glass jar until you are ready to use again.

The Angel's Touch

What you will need:

10 drops ylang ylang oil

5 drops rose oil

4 dandelion flowers

1 teaspoon almond oil

1 teaspoon coconut oil

Directions:

Heat ¼ cup water on the stove until hot, but not boiling. Soak the flowers in this water for 5 minutes.

You can strain out the flowers if you like, or you can leave them in... it's really up to you. I prefer to take them out, as they tend to get too soggy if I don't use all of the treatment at one time, but if you don't mind, leave them in.

Combine the rest of the ingredients in with the water, and carefully stir. You want them all to be as mixed as possible.

Let the mix cool until it is warm, then apply generously to your skin. Massage in and leave on or rinse off.

Store any leftover treatment in an airtight glass jar until you are ready to use again.

The Upside Down

What you will need:

10 drops myrrh oil

5 drops patchouli oil

1 teaspoon organic dried peppermint leaves

1 teaspoon almond oil

1 teaspoon coconut oil

Directions:

Heat ¼ cup water on the stove until hot, but not boiling. Soak the leaves in this water for 5 minutes.

You can strain out the leaves if you like, or you can leave them in... it's really up to you. I prefer to take them out, as they tend to get too soggy if I don't use all of the treatment at one time, but if you don't mind, leave them in.

Combine the rest of the ingredients in with the water, and carefully stir. You want them all to be as mixed as possible.

Let the mix cool until it is warm, then apply generously to your skin. Massage in and leave on or rinse off.

Store any leftover treatment in an airtight glass jar until you are ready to use again.

The Clean and Clear

What you will need:

10 drops rosewood oil

5 drops neroli oil

1 teaspoon organic dried peppermint leaves

1 teaspoon organic dried spearmint leaves

1 teaspoon almond oil

1 teaspoon coconut oil

Directions:

Heat ¼ cup water on the stove until hot, but not boiling. Soak the leaves in this water for 5 minutes.

You can strain out the leaves if you like, or you can leave them in... it's really up to you. I prefer to take them out, as they tend to get too soggy if I don't use all of the treatment at one time, but if you don't mind, leave them in.

Combine the rest of the ingredients in with the water, and carefully stir. You want them all to be as mixed as possible.

Let the mix cool until it is warm, then apply generously to your skin. Massage in and leave on or rinse off.

Store any leftover treatment in an airtight glass jar until you are ready to use again.

Chapter 2 – Dry Skin Solutions You Can't Turn Down

Touch of Moisture

What you will need:

10 drops bergamot oil

5 drops tea tree oil

1 teaspoon dried organic elder flower leaves

1 teaspoon almond oil

1 teaspoon coconut oil

Directions:

Heat ¼ cup water on the stove until hot, but not boiling. Soak the leaves in this water for 5 minutes.

You can strain out the leaves if you like, or you can leave them in... it's really up to you. I prefer to take them out, as they tend to get too soggy if I don't use all of the treatment at one time, but if you don't mind, leave them in.

Combine the rest of the ingredients in with the water, and carefully stir. You want them all to be as mixed as possible.

Let the mix cool until it is warm, then apply generously to your skin. Massage in and leave on or rinse off.

Store any leftover treatment in an airtight glass jar until you are ready to use again.

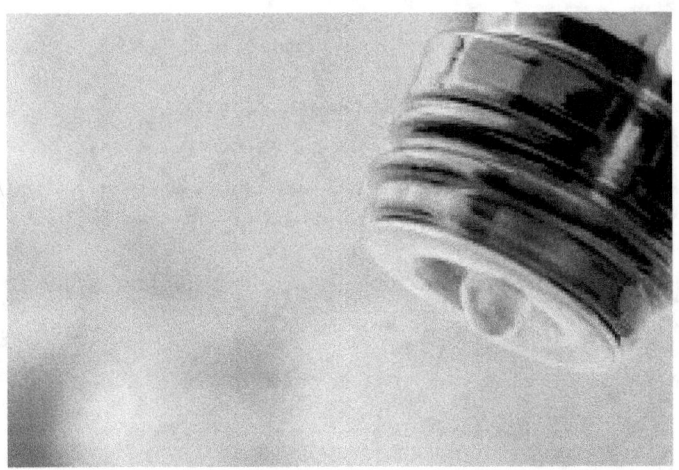

The Perfect Plush

What you will need:

10 drops blue tansy oil

5 drops rose oil

1 teaspoon dried burdock leaves

1 teaspoon almond oil

1 teaspoon coconut oil

Directions:

Heat ¼ cup water on the stove until hot, but not boiling. Soak the leaves in this water for 5 minutes.

You can strain out the leaves if you like, or you can leave them in... it's really up to you. I prefer to take them out, as they tend to get too soggy if I don't use all of the treatment at one time, but if you don't mind, leave them in.

Combine the rest of the ingredients in with the water, and carefully stir. You want them all to be as mixed as possible.

Let the mix cool until it is warm, then apply generously to your skin. Massage in and leave on or rinse off.

Store any leftover treatment in an airtight glass jar until you are ready to use again.

Snowflake Solutions

What you will need:

10 drops myrrh oil

5 drops manuka oil

1 teaspoon dried violet flowers

1 teaspoon almond oil

1 teaspoon coconut oil

Directions:

Heat ¼ cup water on the stove until hot, but not boiling. Soak the flowers in this water for 5 minutes.

You can strain out the flowers if you like, or you can leave them in... it's really up to you. I prefer to take them out, as they tend to get too soggy if I don't use all of the treatment at one time, but if you don't mind, leave them in.

Combine the rest of the ingredients in with the water, and carefully stir. You want them all to be as mixed as possible.

Let the mix cool until it is warm, then apply generously to your skin. Massage in and leave on or rinse off.

Store any leftover treatment in an airtight glass jar until you are ready to use again.

Kiss of the Rose

What you will need:

10 drops rose oil

5 drops bergamot oil

1 teaspoon dried rose petals

1 teaspoon dried crushed rose hips

1 teaspoon almond oil

1 teaspoon coconut oil

Directions:

Heat ¼ cup water on the stove until hot, but not boiling. Soak the hips and petals in this water for 5 minutes.

You can strain out the hips and petals if you like, or you can leave them in... it's really up to you. I prefer to take them out, as they tend to get too soggy if I don't use all of the treatment at one time, but if you don't mind, leave them in.

Combine the rest of the ingredients in with the water, and carefully stir. You want them all to be as mixed as possible.

Let the mix cool until it is warm, then apply generously to your skin. Massage in and leave on or rinse off.

Store any leftover treatment in an airtight glass jar until you are ready to use again.

The Queen Bee

What you will need:

10 drops tea tree oil

5 drops geranium oil

1 teaspoon organic dried crushed plantain

1 teaspoon almond oil

1 teaspoon coconut oil

Directions:

Heat ¼ cup water on the stove until hot, but not boiling. Soak the leaves in this water for 5 minutes.

You can strain out the leaves if you like, or you can leave them in... it's really up to you. I prefer to take them out, as they tend to get too soggy if I don't use all of the treatment at one time, but if you don't mind, leave them in.

Combine the rest of the ingredients in with the water, and carefully stir. You want them all to be as mixed as possible.

Let the mix cool until it is warm, then apply generously to your skin. Massage in and leave on or rinse off.

Store any leftover treatment in an airtight glass jar until you are ready to use again.

Chapter 3 – All Natural Breakout Care

The Prom Queen

What you will need:

10 drops clary sage oil

5 drops eucalyptus oil

1 teaspoon dried organic plantain, crushed

1 teaspoon almond oil

1 teaspoon coconut oil

Directions:

Heat ¼ cup water on the stove until hot, but not boiling. Soak the leaves in this water for 5 minutes.

You can strain out the leaves if you like, or you can leave them in... it's really up to you. I prefer to take them out, as they tend to get too soggy if I don't use all of the treatment at one time, but if you don't mind, leave them in.

Combine the rest of the ingredients in with the water, and carefully stir. You want them all to be as mixed as possible.

Let the mix cool until it is warm, then apply generously to your skin. Massage in and leave on or rinse off.

Store any leftover treatment in an airtight glass jar until you are ready to use again.

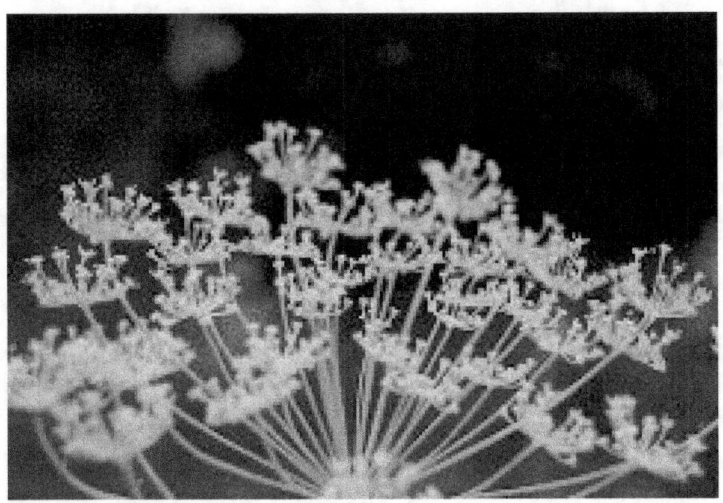

The Lady Luck

What you will need:

10 drops juniper berry oil

5 drops lavender oil

1 teaspoon organic witch hazel bark, crushed

1 teaspoon almond oil

1 teaspoon coconut oil

Directions:

Heat ¼ cup water on the stove until hot, but not boiling. Soak the bark in this water for 5 minutes.

You can strain out the bark if you like, or you can leave them in… it's really up to you. I prefer to take them out, as they tend to get too soggy if I don't use all of the treatment at one time, but if you don't mind, leave them in.

Combine the rest of the ingredients in with the water, and carefully stir. You want them all to be as mixed as possible.

Let the mix cool until it is warm, then apply generously to your skin. Massage in and leave on or rinse off.

Store any leftover treatment in an airtight glass jar until you are ready to use again.

Happy-Go-Lucky

What you will need:

10 drops lemon oil

5 drops lemongrass oil

4 dandelion flowers

1 teaspoon almond oil

1 teaspoon coconut oil

Directions:

Heat ¼ cup water on the stove until hot, but not boiling. Soak the flowers in this water for 5 minutes.

You can strain out the flowers if you like, or you can leave them in... it's really up to you. I prefer to take them out, as they tend to get too soggy if I don't use all of the treatment at one time, but if you don't mind, leave them in.

Combine the rest of the ingredients in with the water, and carefully stir. You want them all to be as mixed as possible.

Let the mix cool until it is warm, then apply generously to your skin. Massage in and leave on or rinse off.

Store any leftover treatment in an airtight glass jar until you are ready to use again.

Princess Pretty

What you will need:

10 drops sandalwood oil

5 drops tea tree oil

1 teaspoon crushed dried rose hips

1 teaspoon almond oil

1 teaspoon coconut oil

Directions:

Heat ¼ cup water on the stove until hot, but not boiling. Soak the rose hips in this water for 5 minutes.

You can strain out the rose hips if you like, or you can leave them in… it's really up to you. I prefer to take them out, as they tend to get too soggy if I don't use all of the treatment at one time, but if you don't mind, leave them in.

Combine the rest of the ingredients in with the water, and carefully stir. You want them all to be as mixed as possible.

Let the mix cool until it is warm, then apply generously to your skin. Massage in and leave on or rinse off.

Store any leftover treatment in an airtight glass jar until you are ready to use again.

Blackhead Banisher

What you will need:

10 drops eucalyptus oil

5 drops geranium oil

1 teaspoon crushed dried organic apricot pit

1 teaspoon almond oil

1 teaspoon coconut oil

Directions:

Heat ¼ cup water on the stove until hot, but not boiling. Soak the pits in this water for 5 minutes.

You can strain out the pits if you like, or you can leave them in... it's really up to you. I prefer to take them out, as they tend to get too soggy if I don't use all of the treatment at one time, but if you don't mind, leave them in.

Combine the rest of the ingredients in with the water, and carefully stir. You want them all to be as mixed as possible.

Let the mix cool until it is warm, then apply generously to your skin. Massage in and leave on or rinse off.

Store any leftover treatment in an airtight glass jar until you are ready to use again.

Chapter 4 – That Youthful Glow

The Ageless Mistress

What you will need:

10 drops frankincense oil

5 drops myrrh oil

1 teaspoon dried rose petals

1 teaspoon dried rose hips

1 teaspoon almond oil

1 teaspoon coconut oil

Directions:

Heat ¼ cup water on the stove until hot, but not boiling. Soak the hips and petals in this water for 5 minutes.

You can strain out the hips and petals if you like, or you can leave them in… it's really up to you. I prefer to take them out, as they tend to get too soggy if I don't use all of the treatment at one time, but if you don't mind, leave them in.

Combine the rest of the ingredients in with the water, and carefully stir. You want them all to be as mixed as possible.

Let the mix cool until it is warm, then apply generously to your skin. Massage in and leave on or rinse off.

Store any leftover treatment in an airtight glass jar until you are ready to use again.

The Youthful Goddess

What you will need:

10 drops jasmine oil

5 drops lavender oil

1 teaspoon dried yarrow leaves

1 teaspoon almond oil

1 teaspoon coconut oil

Directions:

Heat ¼ cup water on the stove until hot, but not boiling. Soak the leaves in this water for 5 minutes.

You can strain out the leaves if you like, or you can leave them in... it's really up to you. I prefer to take them out, as they tend to get too soggy if I don't use all of the treatment at one time, but if you don't mind, leave them in.

Combine the rest of the ingredients in with the water, and carefully stir. You want them all to be as mixed as possible.

Let the mix cool until it is warm, then apply generously to your skin. Massage in and leave on or rinse off.

Store any leftover treatment in an airtight glass jar until you are ready to use again.

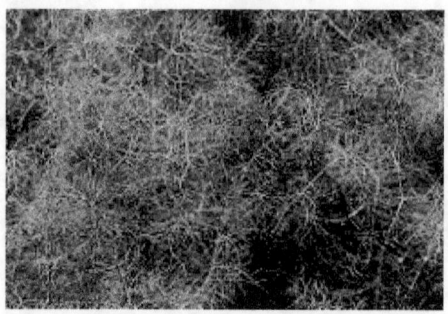

The Elegant Smooth Skinned Maiden

What you will need:

10 drops rose oil

5 drops roman chamomile

1 teaspoon dried calendula petals

1 teaspoon almond oil

1 teaspoon coconut oil

Directions:

Heat ¼ cup water on the stove until hot, but not boiling. Soak the petals in this water for 5 minutes.

You can strain out the petals if you like, or you can leave them in... it's really up to you. I prefer to take them out, as they tend to get too soggy if I don't use all of the treatment at one time, but if you don't mind, leave them in.

Combine the rest of the ingredients in with the water, and carefully stir. You want them all to be as mixed as possible.

Let the mix cool until it is warm, then apply generously to your skin. Massage in and leave on or rinse off.

Store any leftover treatment in an airtight glass jar until you are ready to use again.

The Wrinkle Eraser

What you will need:

10 drops myrrh oil

5 drops frankincense oil

1 teaspoon organic thyme

1 teaspoon organic parsley leaves

1 teaspoon almond oil

1 teaspoon coconut oil

Directions:

Heat ¼ cup water on the stove until hot, but not boiling. Soak the leaves in this water for 5 minutes.

You can strain out the leaves if you like, or you can leave them in... it's really up to you. I prefer to take them out, as they tend to get too soggy if I don't use all of the treatment at one time, but if you don't mind, leave them in.

Combine the rest of the ingredients in with the water, and carefully stir. You want them all to be as mixed as possible.

Let the mix cool until it is warm, then apply generously to your skin. Massage in and leave on or rinse off.

Store any leftover treatment in an airtight glass jar until you are ready to use again.

The Perfectionista

What you will need:

10 drops sandalwood oil

5 drops grapefruit oil

1 teaspoon dried organic lemon zest

1 teaspoon dried organic orange zest

1 teaspoon almond oil

1 teaspoon coconut oil

Directions:

Heat ¼ cup water on the stove until hot, but not boiling. Soak the zest in this water for 5 minutes.

You can strain out the zest if you like, or you can leave them in... it's really up to you. I prefer to take them out, as they tend to get too soggy if I don't use all of the treatment at one time, but if you don't mind, leave them in.

Combine the rest of the ingredients in with the water, and carefully stir. You want them all to be as mixed as possible.

Let the mix cool until it is warm, then apply generously to your skin. Massage in and leave on or rinse off.

Store any leftover treatment in an airtight glass jar until you are ready to use again.

Chapter 5 – The Best of the Rest

The Cheery Eyed

What you will need:

10 drops grapefruit oil

5 drops orange oil

1 teaspoon grapefruit zest

1 teaspoon almond oil

1 teaspoon coconut oil

Directions:

Heat ¼ cup water on the stove until hot, but not boiling. Soak the zest in this water for 5 minutes.

You can strain out the zest if you like, or you can leave them in... it's really up to you. I prefer to take them out, as they tend to get too soggy if I don't use all of the treatment at one time, but if you don't mind, leave them in.

Combine the rest of the ingredients in with the water, and carefully stir. You want them all to be as mixed as possible.

Let the mix cool until it is warm, then apply generously to your skin. Massage in and leave on or rinse off.

Store any leftover treatment in an airtight glass jar until you are ready to use again.

The Fairy Skin

What you will need:

10 drops manuka oil

5 drops blue tansy oil

1 teaspoon dried organic lavender leaves

1 teaspoon dried lemongrass

1 teaspoon almond oil

1 teaspoon coconut oil

Directions:

Heat ¼ cup water on the stove until hot, but not boiling. Soak the leaves in this water for 5 minutes.

You can strain out the leaves if you like, or you can leave them in... it's really up to you. I prefer to take them out, as they tend to get too soggy if I don't use all of the treatment at one time, but if you don't mind, leave them in.

Combine the rest of the ingredients in with the water, and carefully stir. You want them all to be as mixed as possible.

Let the mix cool until it is warm, then apply generously to your skin. Massage in and leave on or rinse off.

Store any leftover treatment in an airtight glass jar until you are ready to use again.

The Sunshine Blast

What you will need:

10 drops geranium oil

5 drops roman chamomile oil

4 dandelion flowers

1 teaspoon almond oil

1 teaspoon coconut oil

Directions:

Heat ¼ cup water on the stove until hot, but not boiling. Soak the flowers in this water for 5 minutes.

You can strain out the flowers if you like, or you can leave them in... it's really up to you. I prefer to take them out, as they tend to get too soggy if I don't use all of the treatment at one time, but if you don't mind, leave them in.

Combine the rest of the ingredients in with the water, and carefully stir. You want them all to be as mixed as possible.

Let the mix cool until it is warm, then apply generously to your skin. Massage in and leave on or rinse off.

Store any leftover treatment in an airtight glass jar until you are ready to use again.

The Graceful Glow

What you will need:

10 drops tea tree oil

5 drops lavender oil

1 teaspoon dried peppermint leaves

1 teaspoon dried organic thyme

1 teaspoon almond oil

1 teaspoon coconut oil

Directions:

Heat ¼ cup water on the stove until hot, but not boiling. Soak the leaves in this water for 5 minutes.

You can strain out the leaves if you like, or you can leave them in... it's really up to you. I prefer to take them out, as they tend to get too soggy if I don't use all of the treatment at one time, but if you don't mind, leave them in.

Combine the rest of the ingredients in with the water, and carefully stir. You want them all to be as mixed as possible.

Let the mix cool until it is warm, then apply generously to your skin. Massage in and leave on or rinse off.

Store any leftover treatment in an airtight glass jar until you are ready to use again.

The Flushed Diva

What you will need:

10 drops ylang ylang oil

5 drops sandalwood oil

1 teaspoon dried organic rose hips, crushed

1 teaspoon witch hazel bark, crushed

1 teaspoon almond oil

1 teaspoon coconut oil

Directions:

Heat ¼ cup water on the stove until hot, but not boiling. Soak the hips and bark in this water for 5 minutes.

You can strain out the hips and bark if you like, or you can leave them in... it's really up to you. I prefer to take them out, as they tend to get too soggy if I don't use all of the treatment at one time, but if you don't mind, leave them in.

Combine the rest of the ingredients in with the water, and carefully stir. You want them all to be as mixed as possible.

Let the mix cool until it is warm, then apply generously to your skin. Massage in and leave on or rinse off.

Store any leftover treatment in an airtight glass jar until you are ready to use again.

Conclusion

There you have it. Everything you need to know to make your own skin care products and keep your skin feeling as flawless and moisturized as you can imagine.

You can rest easy knowing that you are only using the best products on your body, and your health is going to reflect these choices. No matter what, your skin is going to thank you for the hard work you put into keeping it everything it can be, and you are going to feel better for it.

Have fun with these recipes and indulge whenever you feel like you want that little boost. There's no way you can go wrong with your very own skin care regime, and the more you care for your skin, the better off you are going to be.

Say goodbye to the breakouts, the wrinkles, the acne, and the dry, cracked skin as you dive into a fresh new world of healthy living. There's no end to the ways you can care for the skin you live in, and when you make your own products, you are getting the best of the best, every time.

So go ahead and indulge yourself. You know you deserve it.

FREE Bonus Reminder

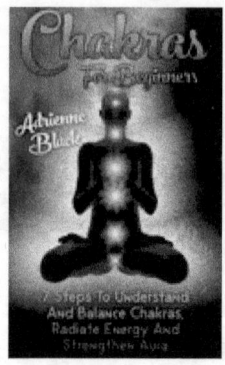

If you have not grabbed it yet, please go ahead and download your special bonus E book *"Chakras for Beginners. 7 Steps To Understand And Balance Chakras, Radiate Energy, And Strengthen Aura"*.

Simply Click the Button Below

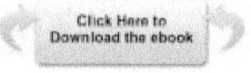

OR Go to This Page

http://lifehacksworld.com/free

BONUS #2: More Free & Discounted Books & Products

Do you want to receive more Free/Discounted Books or Products?

We have a mailing list where we send out our new Books or Products when they go free or with a discount on Amazon. Click on the link below to sign up for Free & Discount Book & Product Promotions.

=> **Sign Up for Free & Discount Book & Product Promotions** <=

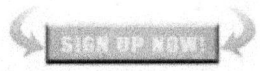

OR Go to this URL

http://zbit.ly/1WBb1Ek

www.ingramcontent.com/pod-product-compliance
Lightning Source LLC
Chambersburg PA
CBHW061931280526
45787CB00004B/1569